Advance Praise

"This book is a wonderful affirmation of what nurturing and believing in yourself can accomplish. For those experiencing difficulties in their lives, Eleanor Miller uses experiences from her own life as she explains the causes of her struggles and the techniques she used in order to heal afterward. It is an extremely interesting and easy read. I could not put it down as it can speak to many. Her experience and insight will truly be a comfort for anyone going through the pain of being selfless and putting themselves last in their own lives. I highly recommend!"

- Lorraine J.

"As a mental health professional for the last 16 years, I know only too well the many complex struggles individuals face. Attempting to overcome obstacles can cause you to become paralyzed. Eleanor's memoir is courageous, inspirational and indeed strong. We all can relate to hitting brick walls and the strength needed to break them down. We all can relate to breaking barriers and getting out of our own way to achieve success. This book will become a staple in my practice as a tool to assist my clientele in their desired growth."

- C. Dacosta, LMSW, CCH, RM

T0159965

"By allowing us to see into her own life stories, she enables us to contemplate our own life struggles and coping abilities. I read it at one sitting and would highly recommend it to anyone who would like to, or needs to, find encouragement."

- Maureen Uniszkiewicz

"The introspection and bravery that shows through on the page should make even the most guarded of us reach inside ourselves."

- Brian Katcher

"Eleanor is a perfectly imperfect person. Her awareness of her own flaws and weaknesses is her biggest virtue and strength, which allows her to continue growing spiritually and emotionally. She has dedicated her life to helping others, from working in the medical field, to helping people spiritually and now as an author. In her book, *If I am So Strong, Why do I feel So Weak?*, she gives us personal insights into her life, her struggles and the changes that she's had to make to grow and overcome her obstacles.

"If you are looking for a straightforward and uncomplicated approach to self-awareness, I recommend Eleanor's book. Let someone who is passionate about helping others be your guide in finding the light at the end of your tunnel."

- Cristina Lijo

"In *If I am so Strong, Why do I Feel So Weak?*, Eleanor Miller uses her own astute self-awareness to help others break down the barriers in their own lives. As a clinical hypnotherapist I see many people who need a boost in confidence in order to achieve their goals. This is an empowering book, that I highly recommend and will help you get the self-confidence you deserve!"

- Dr. Steve G. Jones, Ed.D., Clinical Hypnotherapist

If I'm So Strong,
Why Do I Feel So Weak?

IF I'M SO **STRONG,** WHY DO' I FEEL SO WEAK?

Helping Those Who Help Others
Help Themselves

ELEANOR J. MILLER

NEW YORK

LONDON • NASHVILLE • MELBOURNE • VANCOUVER

If I'm So Strong, Why Do I Feel So Weak?

Helping Those Who Help Others Help Themselves

Published in New York, New York, by Morgan James Publishing in partnership with Difference Press. Morgan James is a trademark of Morgan James, LLC. www.MorganJamesPublishing.com

The Morgan James Speakers Group can bring authors to your live event. For more information or to book an event visit The Morgan James Speakers Group at www.TheMorganJamesSpeakersGroup.com.

ISBN 9781683506430 paperback
ISBN 9781683506447 eBook
Library of Congress Control Number: 2017909835

Cover Design by:
Rachel Lopez
www.r2cdesign.com

Interior Design by:
Chris Treccani
www.3dogcreative.net

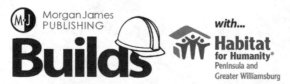

In an effort to support local communities, raise awareness and funds, Morgan James Publishing donates a percentage of all book sales for the life of each book to Habitat for Humanity Peninsula and Greater Williamsburg.

Get involved today! Visit
www.MorganJamesBuilds.com

Dedication

For my daughter, Taylor, my cheerleader throughout this process. I am who I am and have accomplished so much because of you.

Table of Contents

Introduction

Finding Your Authority

"No one can make you feel inferior without your consent"

-Eleanor Roosevelt

I have found through my process of helping others, that there are so many who feel self-doubt when it comes to doing for themselves. It is my hope, for you, as the reader, to see that there is always help and hope for change within you. No matter your situation. This book is geared toward those who have chosen to complete their life of self-sacrifice with their work, such as my brothers and sisters in the Emergency Medical Services. It is my wish to show you that you can help others while helping yourself.

From the moment you were born, people have given you the labels of who you were to be. These labels were usually given with the best intentions. Add to that, the nature of the environment which you were born into and there you have your angst.

You then tried to live up to the expectations given to you by your parents, teachers, siblings, as well as the others who were around you, in your formative years. No wonder you feel so screwed up. Such an overwhelming ebb and flow of emotions brought on by those well-intentioned people. You were and maybe still are, constantly hearing things such as, "You do not want to do that" or, "That would be nice". Or how about, "Hey, you are getting fatter than me, you are too skinny, you are lazy, amazing, or helpful". You were always taught that self-sacrifice is the best label to have and often you find yourself working as a rescuer for the rest of the world.

You have been saving the rest of the world; so, why does it not always feel good for you? You feel great while doing for everyone else but, when it comes to taking care of you, you have no clue. At times, you may have thoughts of being selfish, but it leads to self-chastising, not liking what you are thinking as it goes against your teachings. You may even find that you shut down all your emotions completely. Why? Because, to live up to your given persona, you believe that you are supposed to be there for everyone else, but not yourself. So much so, that you cannot even look inside your dreams or wants anymore; they have all disappeared.

So strong and capable for others, yet so weak for you. Often feeling like no one is there when you need an ear to listen, or a hand for help. You have become the caretaker for everyone! So, where does that leave you? You may even find that you have become a little bitter or have begun not trusting people. Whose fault is it really? You have allowed everything in your life to happen as it did. You have set no boundaries. You secretly long for another life. A life where someone just comes in and takes over the part of taking care of you. With that, you can just go on taking care of everyone else, not needing to change a thing.

Look at what a wonderful person you have become, so caring, strong, nurturing and empathetic, always there for everyone. Giving everyone the time of day but what about you?

What most people do not realize or perhaps see, is that you are hurting just as much and sometimes even more than they can ever imagine. That is because you have become a master of suppressing your emotions. The King or Queen of shutting them down, or ignoring them, because in your mind, you are not as important as others. Or just maybe because you are tired of defending yourself for having them. Besides, it hurts much less this way. Anyway, as you believe, there is a greater good that you should be working on instead of all this trivial stuff.

In life, you were taught and hold firmly in your beliefs, that it is better to give than to receive. This being your truth means that everyone else that ever is or was, is more deserving than you. Turn the other cheek has become your mantra, as well as blessed are the meek, for they shall inherit the earth. You can wait for your just reward! Patience, Love, and Compassion are the end all be all for all, no matter what the cost may be.

There is so much going on in this world now that all these feelings of inadequacy need to stop. You need to realize that only when you help yourself can you better help others. Charity begins in the home; but realize, you are your home. There are more than enough people tearing each other down. You do not need to be one of those who illegitimately tears yourself down. You may feel judged, embarrassed, and alone. You may even wear a mask of happiness and have an excuse ready for why it is not. Of course, you may look good to your family and friends, because to them, you seem to have your life in order. But have you really let them in? Why not? It may be because every time in the past when you have tried to let someone in, they looked at you and had no clue as to what to do. They couldn't handle it. They may have even ignored you or made excuses for not being there. There was one person who once said to me, "You are my rock! If you fall apart what happens to me?" So then, with that said, who is there for you?

Your self-confidence wanes, your self-motivation is nonexistent. You may even become depressed. You let everyone walk over you, often saying to yourself, "why bother"? I am not strong enough or worthy enough to fight for me. You may even fall into the trap of believing that others do not see you as important, therefore, neither do you.

You are great at consoling others and giving advice. But you take none of your own. Are you happy? Work sucks at times, because you allow everyone to bulldoze you. You try not to cause any upsets. Boundaries are nonexistent. You give and give till there is nothing left to give and then you give some more. You then may even try to take on more and then spiral out of control.

You do deserve all that is good and happy. You do deserve abundance and you *are* the authority of your life. You find that you cannot change the way of others. What is your typical response? You try to change who you are to make them happy.

It seems though, that they keep wanting more and more and then, when you finally get the momentum of their rules, of their wants and needs, they go and change them on you! Why, oh why, do you allow this?

You need to believe in you. You are stronger than you know and it is all inside. Why do you think the law of abundance does not work for you? Could be, deep down you really do not believe that you are deserving? The mind is a most powerful thing. I like to think of it as a computer. Always remembering all the programming entered into it. It remembers every little detail of every part of your life, including your actions and reactions. Without you even realizing, your mind is doing the reacting for you, based on what the computer has stored from your past.

Oftentimes, you have no clue as to the why when you are reacting to a situation. You then feel the need to look for the why. When an answer is received as to that why, you question it. And so on, and so on, and so on. STOP! Get off the never-ending ride of doubting yourself. It is not working! Take off your mask and be the real you that you were meant to be. The you that you agreed to be. Take life as a lesson and see things for how they really are.

You cannot change people and you should not let them change you. Do not be afraid, for what is the worst possible thing that can happen? You may be in the same spot you are in. But, the best thing that can happen, is you find you! Besides, are these people really looking out for your best interest? Love yourself first and that is where the happiness lies. It is within you. It is you. I can say this; because I have been there and never thought I would be able to see that light at the end of the tunnel.

Here is a page from an old journal that I found recently. This was from a time when I was questioning myself and who I was.

"I need to believe in myself somehow. I mean I am a good person, I have a very good work ethic and I am always there for others. I have always dreamt of helping people and I now work in an emergency system where I can help people who are at their worst and sometimes get to see the best in people. I love when I can help them to find hope and strength or give needed compassion to their emergent problem. I genuinely love my job and would not trade it for the world. I have helped people who were ready to end their life and have brought them to the place of seeing that proverbial light at the end of the tunnel. I cried with them as they hugged me and thanked me for saving their life and for giving them hope. I have seen people who were dying and so afraid, and after being with them they thanked me for comforting them. I have also brought new life into this world.

I do have respect from my coworkers for the job I do and from most of my patients, even if they were the nastiest people. Many have come to trust me and let me in. I can get most people to trust me. I take care of everyone from my husband, my children, an older brother who had a terrible accident as well as all the people who call for help and yet I feel so alone.

Why is it then, I don't ask for help when it comes to my personal life? I do not want to bother people with my problems; they have enough of their own issues. Besides, I am a strong person and should be able to do it on my own. I don't like to take advantage of anyone. I don't know what is wrong with me. I can help everyone else but when it comes to me and my problems, I feel like there must be something wrong with me. I am embarrassed to ask for help.

Sometimes I believe that I am not good enough for my husband, as he can't understand why I can never get everything done. I feel like I am constantly doing, but it is never enough. I mean I get the kids up for school, have breakfast with them, go over their homework, get them on the bus, do for my brother his physical therapy, mow the lawn if needed, vacuum the house, make dinner for them so that it only needs to be reheated, take my shower and go to work by 2pm. I know that I need to change things but I don't know if I can, and I don't know how. Deep down, I know I am doing a lot and yet, I feel like I am not doing enough. To change things might create more chaos, and I need to just calm things down and make everyone happy. I am strong for everyone else, but I do not know what to do for me. Maybe I am just overthinking all of this. There are times when I think I should leave but then I don't know if I could make it on my own. Who would help me? Mom and Dad are gone! No family nearby; his parents are why he is the way he is and I do not want them around the kids so much. What would people think? What about my kids? I would be a failure, I made a vow and just must suck it up, for better or worse like they say. I guess I got worse. Life is not supposed to be easy anyway so, why am I whining? I wish I could just run away where no one knows me and begin a new life!"

These were all the things that went through my head for the longest time. For too long!

I am writing all this and putting myself out there, so that I may show you through my experiences, that yes, you have the power and are more than capable of making your life filled with blue skies and peace. You can push away the gray clouds of doubt and fear that sometimes override your every move; you just need to let it in. Easier said than done, I get that, especially if you tend to rule with your conscious mind of logical thinking and skepticism.

I believe that we as society have been taught only one way of thinking, so that we may conform, to fit in, so to speak. I believe that we are ruled by EGO and by that I do not mean in a narcissistic way, but in a way where with human conditioning throughout the ages we have allowed ourselves to believe that we are small and unworthy. This has only taken away our confidence and belief in ourselves. It is this thinking which has caused us to lose our connectedness to all that we have within us and are deserving of.

I have made it my purpose in this life to help you see that you can move away from this chaotic world of negative reactions and manipulations. With that, you will find the strength that is inside you, and then comes a real inner peace. This peace is within each one of us. Many speak of this inner peace and strength, but either don't show the way, or when they do, they believe their way is the only way.

I know who I thought I was, but more importantly, I know who I really am now. I know that we all are born with the same birthrights, which we have learned throughout the ages to push away with such ease.

I have been through many traumas throughout my life and lost myself for so long. I believe we are put here to find our connection to one another and for us to realize that we are all deserving of joy and abundance. The only way that we can find it is through ourselves. It is within all of us! Game on! Let me show you how you matter and let you know that you can find your authority for yourself. Most importantly, you can find it in a way that is comfortable for you. This finding will benefit both you and those around you!

Chapter 1

What is Your Faction?

"Categorical labeling is a tool that humans use to resolve the impossible complexity of the environments we grapple to perceive."
- Adam Alter from *Psychology Today*

Labels, labels, labels! I believe that everyone has at least two and sometimes many more. You were given labels and have carried them with you since early childhood!

You see, your labels are lovingly given to you when you are first born. Your parents, grandparents, siblings, family and friends all are so willing to partake in this ancient pastime. These labels may begin with being gender specific and then move onto personality characteristics. Anything you do that goes against these labels may be perceived as you acting in a negative way.

It appears that humanity has always liked to put people into categories. This is a tradition that was passed down for generations and is still going strong. The attraction about labeling is it is believed to be your truth. It is supposed to make life so much easier for you and those you first meet. It makes life easier for you, because you now know who people expect you to be. These labels also allow others to know exactly who you are, as well as let them know your strengths and weaknesses. How wonderful for society to pass down, from the first generation to our time now, this way of categorizing through labels. It has allowed us to conform and be who and what we are meant to be.

As per the bible, Cain and Abel were the first generation born into humanity. They were given labels of evil, self-centered, good, loving, slacker, hard worker, instigator and peacemaker. Even though we have never met them, we know who they are and what they were all about through their labeling. You see now how easy it is for all those you meet, to know who you are prior to getting to even meet you! Just by learning of your labels through family, friends, and coworkers.

We have been taught who we are through our gender labels. How wonderfully easy this makes it for both women and men. With our labels come attached duties or actions so that we always know the roles we need to play. The men are the hunters, warriors, the stronger sex. The women who are weaker physically and mentally, need to do only the soft and tender things. Men are the fixers and women are the boo-boo kissers and peacemakers. Add to that your personality labels and characterizations and there you stand, transparent and clear for all the world to see.

Society in its many ways still holds true to this pastime. When meeting someone new, we all have the belief that we know who the person is prior to our meeting just from the many labels we have heard that were given to them. For example, all someone needs to say about me is, meet Eleanor, Chick's daughter. Voila! His friends may feel like they instantly know me from the labels they have heard I have been given.

I hope by now you realize that I am being a bit sarcastic in my approach to how society did and still does us all a favor with categories and labeling. All this categorizing reminds me of the movie Divergent. It is a movie that depicts a society, where once you become of age you are mandated to pick one group to live out the rest of your life with. There are five groups that society deems beneficial and acceptable for you to choose from. The one which you were born into and four others. You do not know much about the other groups, but a mind test is performed on you and tells you which group you would fit into the most, per your thoughts and beliefs. Once a specific group is picked, you are to take on all the labels, beliefs, and personalities of this group and hold them as your own for the rest of your life. If you should happen to choose to leave your group to go into another, no interaction at all is allowed with old family or friends. Society keeps them unconnected. You are to only be with your kind. There is only one way of thinking, allowing you to fit in always. Only group speak, never straying, never changing, always just being, for fear of becoming an outcast. This is supposed to make life's choices so easy for you, as you have all the answers of how you are to act and think. Any thoughts or actions outside these parameters, or by not choosing a group, makes you an outcast of society! This included having an understanding and some beliefs of all the groups. You are only to act in one way and not be divergent, a free thinker, with individual thoughts.

Trusting no one, never feeling close and always afraid of being judged or deemed as unworthy. I, for one, do see so many similarities between the *fictional* world depicted in the movie and ours. Where individuality can be frowned upon and you can be made to feel like an outcast. Not fitting into any group at all. Do we need to really fit into any one group? Is individualism that bad?

You do have your own unique personality and you are always learning what works or does not work for you. Why then, do your labels never change? You seem to hold onto your labels so tightly and have such fear or guilt when you do not follow through with their dictated actions. You may also find that if a label is stressed by someone which goes against the ones given to you, an instant panic can happen. Action is usually quickly taken to change that *negative* label, to one that is believed to be more fitting, positive and acceptable. Convincing the person involved that even though we may have slipped, that is not who we really are. We want nothing but what society deems as positive. For example, especially for women, if you stress a point on a project while at work, you may be taken as being bossy or bitchy/overly assertive. You do not want to be perceived as being nasty or on the rag, so now you find yourself overcompensating, losing confidence or apologizing for something unnecessarily.

Whew, thank God for labels, for where would you be without them! How would we ever know who we are supposed to be? Caregiver, nurturer, someone who will drop everything for someone, a good student, a good person who helps everyone and speaks for the underdog. She is so quiet and easy to please, she causes no problems and so on and so on. These are the labels that are for the world to see, to show that you do indeed fit into a mold acceptable to all! How amazing you are! How proud you feel to grow up knowing all of this. You believe in these labels with all your being and the world sees you as this!

Just follow me for a few moments and imagine yourself in the following situations. Imagine that your journey of labels began at birth. You are an only girl born into a family with four older brothers. Now, I am almost positive that in this situation, if I ask them, they will say that you are and were so spoiled. It seems most brothers gripe about this consistently from day one until the day you die. But, because you are always hearing this, you have taken on the challenge of disproving this label, by proving yourself consistently in everything you do. You are always proving to yourself and others that you can and will do, without help, the task at hand.

And so, you see yourself growing up in this middle-class family, your father works two jobs to provide all the necessities in life, including a private school education. Your parents do things the best way they know how. Your dad's way is to make you better at everything you do. He understands that you being a female, you need to do certain things in life. His way is to show you what is wrong, so you can fix the problem or situation.

Imagine bringing home your end of the year report card while finishing eighth-grade. You are so proud you brought home three A pluses, one A minus, and the rest regular As with a college reading level. You see yourself running home from school, showing first your mother. She gives you kudos telling you that you should go and show your dad. He of course, is at the bar. It is still early enough, as he is working his part-time job there. He does not drink while working. You run down the block and burst into that bar, so excited to show him what you have accomplished. Reaching for his glasses, he puts them on and studies the report card so carefully. After what seems like forever, you eagerly interrupt his inspection with, "Well, what do you think?" Awaiting a good pat on the back, he turns to you, without even a smile and says, "Why aren't they all A pluses? I know you can do better than this." And now you feel, in that moment, as if all the people in that bar are staring at you. They are giving you the look of, you are such a failure. You are so embarrassed. Talk about feeling instantly defeated and deflated. You believed this would have made him proud. Never thinking anyone could find fault in this. Now, you leave with the feeling of you are not good enough and what is worse is that now everyone knows it.

This causes you to doubt everything you do. It makes you question if you are capable of ever being great. It makes you a thinker of all the possibilities of what may or may not go wrong in any situation which life may offer. Always having to prove yourself and needing to be better than any expectations you could think of. Being number two, or God forbid, number three, is appalling and means you are a failure.

This feeling of having to be perfect started at such a young age. It was even reinforced in school. That private school was going to make you the best you could be! So much pressure to be perfect in everything you do that you passed out in your second-grade class. The sheer fright that came over you when you saw Sister Philemona swinging that yard stick over her head and hitting the student in front of you. He did not know the answer to the question he was asked. You're next in line and doubting yourself, you are not one hundred percent sure. Bam! To the floor! That was so much easier than the berating and beating you would have taken. You do not dare tell your parents about the beatings in school, as you believe that you deserve to be punished for not knowing everything. Psychological warfare at its best and what a good little soldier you are! You can see now, why you would have anxiety when you are put on the spot! You are so afraid of being judged and embarrassed by failure. You are always supposed to be smart and know the answers to everything. To be the one who pleases and not disappoints anyone.

As a young child, you try constantly to please your father. Even though he was mostly unavailable to you. Often coming home drunk, stumbling down the block. Being so young and with your friends, you distracted them away from views of him or put on a smile and made a joke out of it as it tears you up inside. You feel the stares and swear you can hear the judgments, even if it was just in your thoughts. These looks are horrible, they make you believe that they feel sorry for you for having a father like that. If only you could make him happy; he would not drink. Then, he and your mom would get along so much better. They argue so much when he is drunk, which is almost always. You feel stuck in the middle and know in your young mind that there must be something you could do to fix this. There will be a fight in the house tonight. You try protecting your mom by talking to your dad and vice versa. Doesn't always work.

All these labels and categories come with values for you that you need to follow. Always having to be what you are told to be. You find out that you are only human and will never be special or worthy enough. How disappointing to learn as a young child that you will never be humble enough or ever be good enough.

My question for you now, which group do you choose? Do you wish to be the Divergent one? Some people call them outcasts, and then others call them trailblazers. The choice is yours. You can be in a faction or be a trailblazer.

I had a client who I asked this question of. She just looked at me and broke down for a moment. Having grown exhausted of being trapped in a specific group and its predetermined mold was causing her to have a burning desire to break free of the expectations that everyone else has of her. She was always told she was the wild one and capable of getting whatever she wanted. She was tired of living the lie that she outgrew so long ago. She knew deep down that was not how she truly felt, but no one wanted to believe her. She just wanted people to care for her needs and know that she needed tenderness too.

After speaking to her it was easy to see, that she was looking for the tenderness and respect that she felt she never had. Feeling her family life and work were going down the drain. My client had become depressed, not wanting to do anything or be around anyone. Everything seemed like a chore, so much bigger than it should be that it became paralyzing and nothing got done.

I explained to her that I wanted to do a hypnosis session. I could see the fear in her eyes. Firstly, she was afraid of not having control and secondly, believed that she was way too stressed for it to even work. We then discussed her fears of hypnosis and what an actual session entails. It was only when she felt comfortable, we did the session. After that session, I saw the stress level go down tremendously, so much so, she did not want to leave as this was the most relaxed she felt in a long while. At a later time, coming back for a follow up, my client had noticed improvement in her feeling of herself. After a few short sessions she realized that she was holding on to the beliefs of those labels in her mind. She had a hard time letting them go for they had been with her throughout all these years. We did a session of erasing old labels and instilling new and fitting ones for who she is now.

She recently told me how she is doing so much better in work since releasing her need to be perfect in everything that she does. It was negatively affecting her and her coworkers as she was holding everything to the highest standard and nothing less, and had the need to control everyone and everything she did. Her home life too is much improved. She now hears and shares in more laughter from those she loves. Feeling less stressed and more productive, she was amazed that in a short time her life had become happy again.

Who do you want to be?

Here is a little exercise that may help you become who you wish yourself to be. You will need two pieces of paper. On one page write down 'feelings of no use to me' as the title and on the other write 'new and improved me' or 'the real me' whatever resonates with you and what you want to be recognized for as the title.

Now I want you to write down all the labels and feelings you no longer wish to keep in your life anymore. Feelings that you no longer wish to accept. Feelings and labels such as: weak, sadness, self-doubt, un-lovable, not good enough and whatever else it is you feel or believe.

After you are done writing these down, I want you to take your pen/pencil and cross out these words. Really make them disappear from the page. These are no longer accepted in your life. Rip up this page and throw it away as you no longer accept these in your life.

Now on the second piece of paper, I want you to put all the positive traits of you! The real you in a bright color! Make it gold if you can, for you are golden! Write down words like: strong, capable, smart, dynamic, happy, loving to self, loving to others and everything else positive that you can think of. Put this in a place, where you can see it every morning and throughout the day. Remind yourself of who you really are!

Chapter 2

I'm Sorry I'm Such a Biotch

"They'll insult, belittle and criticize you. Sometimes in a teasing/joking way, pushing your boundaries until you finally speak up. Then, they use your reactions to make you seem crazy. They can turn and easy going person into a hot mess of insecurities and self-doubt"

-Author Unknown

Tired of keeping the peace? You must be tired of apologizing for nothing or for everything? What else can you do? You are the peacekeeper for all! You try to keep the peace at home, at work, with friends as well as with all others who you meet. It can be overwhelming. There are times

15

you just want to scream and tell everyone to shut up. All this peacekeeping leaves you exhausted, and at times full of despair. Why is it so draining to be the peacekeeper? Why does it leave you so down and out? I mean, after all, you are following the rules given to you. So, if you are being so good, why are you so unhappy?

Why is it that you feel so afraid to offend someone? You believe in the truth. Is it not said that the truth will set you free? So why is it then, that you cannot follow through with speaking the truth? It is not that you lie, but instead, you say nothing. Is that not the same as not speaking the truth? People are always in search of answers for many things in life, especially of themselves. They will ask questions of you. But it seems that when you tell them something that goes against what they want to hear, you immediately find they are visibly upset. Now, because of your tender heart strings, you try to soften everything and often find yourself apologizing for speaking what you believe to be the truth. You were not nasty in what you said, but it hurt them anyway. Or, you may find at times, that even when you say what you believe to be the right thing, there is resistance the whole way. It seems that some people are great at turning around what you even meant to say. Leaving you puzzled and wondering how the words you said even conveyed a portion of how they were received.

Sometimes it feels like most people are trying to be something greater or at least different than what they are showing themselves to be in their actions. When you see this difference, it becomes difficult to state what you see, for they are not receptive, even when they ask, no matter how softly you may put it. This can cause you to go into a downward spiral of 'I am no good' and cause you to feel guilty for hurting their feelings. People like to use this against you at times. Sometimes knowingly and sometimes without thought, like an automatic reaction. Because you, being good hearted, do not like to see the hurt in others, as you know all too well how it feels. So instead, you try to boost people constantly, feeding their ego even at the cost of yourself. You then find yourself apologizing profusely.

I remember there was a time that I found myself apologizing for a whole week. I was taking my oldest brother Joe, into my home. He was in a terrible accident that left him with a brain injury and multiple physical disabilities. It was my husband Glenn's idea. While in front of my family, he suggested that we take care of him instead of putting him into long term care. Joe had already spent nine months in the hospital and brain rehabilitation. We all knew Joe would do much better in the home environment. Wow, I was taken aback. I thought I would have resistance in even bringing this thought up to my husband.

The only problem now was that things needed to change for this move to happen. We needed to add a bathroom and put walls up before he came.

The rehabilitation people came and told me what exactly was needed to make Joe comfortable. Measurements were taken to make the bathroom accessible as well as making some changes to have a wheelchair capable of going through the rooms. So the renovations that we wanted to save up for and complete down the road, were to be done quickly. Great family project? Not really. Glenn, was not happy with doing any kind of work like that as it always turned into a fiasco. But, maybe this time would be different.

I found myself taking care of my four-year-old son and two-year-old daughter, working my full-time job and putting in a bathroom upstairs. I paid for the plumbers to bring the pipes up, but the funds were low to pay someone to do the sheetrock, spackling and laying of tiles. I researched and learned how to do the tiling. All the while Glenn was reminding me that there was not much time before Joe came home. I felt responsible; after all he is *my* brother.

I took off from work for two days and asked Glenn for his help. His response being, "Someone needs to watch the kids".

"I am sorry you are right", I responded. As I was cutting tiles, I found that my hands were blistered but I felt good as it seemed I was getting the hang of it. After some time, the kids started crying for me; they were hungry. Pissed off because I was trying to get something that needed to be done, done, I asked Glenn to feed them. "But they want you", he stated. I went into the kitchen and made lunch for them, then went back upstairs to finish the tiling. Glenn came upstairs to inspect the progress and proceeded to tell me how I had not spent any time with the kids, and how I was being unfair to them. A discussion ensued and I found myself apologizing for not being there for the kids, making dinner and then getting them ready for bed, while Glenn went out to the store.

The next day, getting ready to go back and finish laying the tiles before I had to go to work, I told Glenn of my plans. Here came the excuse of 'Well, I watched the kids for you yesterday, and I want to go to the store for a few things that I did not get last night". "Well, we do not have time and I need to finish" was my reply. Another discussion that ended with me apologizing and the letting go of the tiling. The next day, I was just waking up and I heard from him, "Well it is not going to get done if WE don't get on it today". If only I could get this right, what is wrong with me? Getting upset, I suggested a sitter for the kids and that got knocked down. How could I inconvenience someone else?

After a week of this back and forth, and being pulled beyond my stretch I became a little cranky. Okay, a lot cranky. I lashed into him telling him that I needed his assistance. He looked at me as he stated something to the fact that he couldn't understand what was wrong with me and asked me why I was acting so nasty. According to him, he had been helping; he was taking care of the kids to give me the time. He even washed the dishes and did a load of laundry for me. Feeling defenseless and guilty because it was my brother, and okay he did do some housework, I apologized for my mood and finished up my project. Now, there was peace in the house! Or was there?

Are you always wrong? Do you apologize for having feelings? Do you apologize for apologizing? At times do you find you are asking yourself, why am I so cranky and needy? Guilt ridden and oh so sorrowful?

I mean, you may start out with a strong feeling of knowing what upset you and feeling honest in your convictions. You decide that you will talk it out with whomever. Only to find yourself, by the end of the conversation, apologizing for even brining the subject up. You have been so turned around, and have no clue as to how that even happened. Now, thinking to yourself, how can I be such an ass? Why do I start trouble? Why can't I just let things be? Always being sorry, having the feeling of what is wrong with you. Can you be that messed up? After all, you just wanted to do the right thing and you always seem to believe you are acting with the best intentions. So, why does it always seem to go in such a different direction when you are only trying to do the right thing for everyone?

I know now that it was I who allowed it. I allowed the manipulation. It was so subtle at first and I had no clue that it was even being done. I understand that it was done in a way which played on my heart strings. I was always a sucker for the victimization role of others. You see, we are people who like to feel needed and as the rescuer we always want to help those who are hurting. It was only after some time that I realized the patterns and began to question how I was always wrong. I tried to speak about it to Glenn, only to have tears from him and more heart strings pulled. It was always about how I was hurting him. I began to realize that I was only valued for what I could do for him!

Constant apologizing and acceptance of guilt caused me to no longer believe in myself. I found myself always sitting on the sidelines and allowing things to happen. I was feeling powerless in my personal life. And now, instead of being loving, kind and caring I was becoming resentful at everyone else for not believing in me. That resentment led to some guilt for becoming angry at those who did not even know the whole story.

I finally decided that I needed to do something for me. I was not close to my family anymore and needed some outside pleasure. I met a woman who owned a beautiful store filled with crystals and books. I loved being in her store and joined her meditation group. She taught me about gratitude. That when someone does something for you, just say "Thank you". She also taught me how to say no confidently.

It needs to be practiced first. She would have me practice in my mind. "You know most of the scenarios", she would say. Say "no" to your manipulator and when asked why, just state, "Because I do not want to", and leave it at that. It does throw them off and they will continue to try the stories to pull your heart strings, she explained. Just keep practicing, standing strong in your mind and stop rewarding the behavior when it happens. With time, change began to happen. This change was a growing confidence of my actions and with that a self-love was growing within me.

I had a client who we will call Carol. Carol came to me because she felt like she could never say no. She was guilt ridden and becoming angry with herself. Her story felt so familiar to me. She lost enjoyment in going to any family functions with her husband. Even gatherings with friends was a chore. She always seemed so drained prior to getting to their destination and often felt guilty if her husband was not enjoying himself, which seemed like always.

Carol also complained of feeling that she needed to do everything. If she made a complaint, she would, after a conversation with her husband, feel like she was so wrong in her judgment.

Right before coming to me, there was an incident that brought her to such a state. She was helping her children with homework as her son had a project due the next day and she had yet to do the dinner dishes as she would have normally done. Her husband mentioned the dishes. She felt like he was upset that they were not done yet. He came in while she was working with her son and told her he had done the dishes. Carol immediately felt bad and guilty and followed with an apology spree. She took his stating he washed the dishes as a negative criticism. She felt he would believe she did not finish her wifely chores and hold it against her because he did something for her.

After the first session, she left feeling calmer and more relaxed about things. After a few weeks, she had such a turn around and now even has a honey-do list for her husband to help with some of the chores around the house. All without guilt, for she believes it to be a partnership now. She came to realize that she is not responsible for everything, including his responses to her. That she needs to be happy in herself and who she is and then she can help those around her. She understands that she has needs and can now ask without feeling that she is being selfish. Her response when someone, especially her husband, does something for her, is now gratitude and not feelings of personal failure. More importantly, she has learned to say no and has gained the confidence of speaking to him about his actions and how they make her feel. They are enjoying going out more and agree on where they wish to go. She is so much happier, and so is her family.

They say what you put out is what you get. Carol is putting out more confidence and respect for herself and is getting that in return, even in work. I find this is important for those who work in rescue situations. When you bring the confidence of yourself to any situation, you can think more clearly and make better decisions.

Chapter 3

How Are You So Good

"There are few good women who don't tire of their role"

-Francoise de La Rochefoucald

You may have been taught to be "perfect", by living your labels and within your groups in life. Always being the good girl. If you are so perfect, why then do you at times feel so doubtful, so disheartened and unable to do for yourself?

Have you become the quiet little church mouse, never speaking your voice? I am not saying your voice needs to be bold or nasty in bringing it out, but do you even put your thoughts or ideas out there anymore? Do you wonder what has become of you? Are there times when you lack confidence and find you are judging yourself so much more? Feeling judged every step of the way? Allowing yourself to be manipulated into doing as others want and need?

There are those who always just accept the status quo. Shutting down all emotions and wants. Because it seems easier to do that than to think of one's ideas or dreams as significant. Many have done it so well, they have no idea anymore of what they even want in life.

Imagine, coming to the point of believing that everyone else is smarter and more intelligent than you, especially in the work that you are doing for them. With that said, let me ask you this, why do you believe they have *you* doing it? Is it because they just needed a person to perform the task that any monkey can do? Or is it because they realize you can accomplish the task at hand? Think hard about that. Even if you knew nothing about the task, you can accomplish the learning process and get it done for them! Is that someone who is not capable? After all, you are trusted to make split second decisions about people's lives every day in work, such as when you do a quick diagnosis and administer life-saving drugs. Drugs that can kill if you are wrong.

There are those who have become numb in thoughts and feelings. Happy to be the doer of other people's plans oftentimes, with never an interjection of something which comes from them. Something which may be better, but, no one will ever know.

I believe that with all we have learned throughout our formative years, one of the most compelling traits we have learned and hold onto for dear life is fear. The fear of being judged is huge. Oh, my God! I cannot do that! What will everyone think?

It is said that we fear not the darkness, for we are comfortable in it, even though it may cause us misery. That is because it is what we know. So, I ask you, is fear of the unknown, of living in your power, what you are really frightened of? Fear of 'What if you stand up for yourself, and upset people'? Fear that you will make changes and be different from who you are expected to be? You may be a bit nervous about all of this and if so, feel it in the pit of your stomach.

Please know, fear caused me to make many mistakes in life as well. There were many times where I wanted to do what I believed to be best for all involved, including me. But the fear stopped me. Finally, I stated NO MORE! And began my journey.

I became defiant in the way of knowing what I wanted to do and trying to take control. I am doing it dammit! But alas, I would feel guilty and the fear of being wrong in what I was doing, stepped in and stopped me. The fear of being wrong and needing concrete proof of anything robbed me of so much happiness. How do you prove feelings/emotions? They are something that you feel. They are hard to explain. And besides, I was already used to knowing that my feelings, per the people I loved, were not always on target.

I feared making boundaries, because I thought I would become a control freak and be the biggest pain in the butt there ever was. I could not even explain what or how I felt. I had become numb to everything and so adept at turning off my emotions. If an emotion ever tried to sneak in, faster than a speeding bullet, I could quickly turn it off. I became everyone's rock because I could be so strong in any situation. I even had the thought that shutting down all emotions was doing tremendous good for me and my family! I believed it would make me feel stronger! After all, I do shut them down while I am working! Why couldn't I do that everywhere else? I could just live my life as if I was only there for others' purposes, and then I would be fulfilling my destiny!

I admit that living a life without fear is not an easy thing to do. It is everywhere you look! From television, newspapers and everything else that is around us. But living a life without the fear of being an individual is freeing and rewarding. Living a life of not doubting yourself, of having confidence and being the you were meant to be is what life is supposed to be.

> *"Why am I letting you comfort me?" He stared over her head.*
> *"Because, I've made sure you have no one else to turn to."*
> **- Kersley Cole, *Lothaire***

Let's see if you can relate to this. You have a strong belief in marriage which is supposed to be one hundred percent give and take by both parties, is it not? Is it supposed to be that you only give and he only takes? What else could it be, because you are realizing that you are manipulated into things that you do not even want? You being such a strong sympathizer, have fallen into allowing the victim role that he plays so well! This role includes things that seem oh so trivial such as picking out a couch, to major life decisions such as naming your daughter.

Why would you continue to allow this? It is the fear of the unknown, of the what-ifs, that keep you in the situation you are in.

Fear is the one distraction that keeps us stagnant and unable to move forward in life. It often paralyzes us from making the decisions we wish to make and therefore keeps us in situations we would rather not be in.

The longer we give credibility to our fear the more complex and compelling it becomes. Living in this constant fear can cause depression, anxiety and self-doubt. We cease to exist as who we are, losing our identity.

We have known fear our whole life. We learned fear from our parents through consequences of our actions in school as well as in our workplace. Fear is so prevalent in the world that we live, and keeps us from accomplishing at times the simplest of tasks.

I worked with someone who was older, in her forties, and was thinking about going to college. She had never even graduated high school, but had eventually gotten her GED. She did not feel smart enough and was afraid of looking the fool, especially if she failed. After a few months of debating this with herself, she decided to go. This decision was not a happy one with her husband. His biggest concern was, he may have to do more duties in the house while she was having fun in school. She made me laugh as she told me about registration day. Here she was having hot flashes from menopause, red face and sweating, while standing with the hormonal eighteen-year-old freshmen, who had just graduated high school. She felt embarrassed initially but stayed in line, while all the flirting and such was going on around her. After standing in line and listening to them, she played in her head our pep talks and decided to become the next brilliant mind.

Her school career began again in a great way. She immersed herself into everything and was not going to miss out on anything. She gave herself the pep talk of how she was here to learn, and being older and wiser, would take advantage of it all. She explained that she always sat herself in the front of class to keep from becoming distracted. That is how serious she was about not letting being scared stop her. English Lit homework, wow. On our down time, she would read a story three times at least to get what the professor was looking for. She was getting the allegory and such, which made her ecstatic. She told me how one day while handing back the homework, her professor read her grade out loud, 105. She was the only one; everyone else had a C or lower, mostly lower. So now all the kids that were flunking were surrounding her and calling her Mrs. 105. They asked her how she did it. After getting over her initial embarrassment, she told them, they needed to do their homework properly which sometimes takes two or three reads of a story. They quickly reminded her that they were too busy going out with friends. They had a life, as they were not married with kids and responsibility.

The next class she found five kids running to her to check their homework, or better yet, to have her give them her answers. After hearing the word "help" she was compelled to help them fix what they did not do.

What ever happened to accountability? She quickly realized what they were doing and it was becoming too much. To avoid saying no, she took her time and came to class just as it was beginning. This way there were no hurt feelings and hopefully, they would learn to be accountable for themselves. This is the only way she knew how to create a boundary and not be manipulated into doing what she did not want to do. She did not want to be in a class where everyone was not liking her because she was doing well, but did not want to give away what she was working for. She did have other responsibilities and they were just out partying. After a few days of doing this one of the other students asked, "why don't you come in early anymore"?

Her reply, "I have responsibilities and yet do what I have to do. You need to do the same." It felt good to say this and she found that some were asking for advice, instead of the answers. She found her way to begin creating her boundaries.

Are you always trying to please everyone and yet always questioning why people take advantage of you?

My client was afraid and almost backed out because of the fear she experienced. Knowing that she would never know if she did not try, she pushed herself and made one of the best decisions in her life. She found out what she was truly capable of and because of this has gained so much more confidence in herself. It did help that she opened up to others, and spoke of her fears. She allowed herself to be vulnerable in admitting that she was afraid, and once she opened, she found people to talk to who cheered her on the whole way.

There is fear at home. Fear of hurting the ones we love. Whether it is because of our dislike of seeing their pain or the fear of being on our own.

We learned fear from our parents, with consequences, from school. Fear is everywhere and there is nowhere to hide from it. What we can change is our response to fear and how we allow or do not allow others to control us with it. One huge problem that so many complain of is work. So many fear retaliation and therefore put up with what seems to be unfair practices and conform just to keep the peace and hopefully their job.

There are many who are in management positions who feel that they are the ultimate authority. And with that authority comes power that to them means dominance, loving to incite fear and dissention. The dissention among the workers gives them total control of your actions.

While on the job, have you ever taken a promotion? Or wanted to? But stopped yourself as it would take you out of the protection of the union. Or more importantly, it would take you away from those you have worked with for so long and have come to think of as family?

You know doing such a thing can cause rifts. Sometimes the crew members who you have worked with for so long will pull away from you. Or you feel you may have to pull away from them. You have been in on the conversations about the other supervisors and see how it is frowned upon to get along with the crews. You almost have to become two faced, and while with management, agree to their faces with what they want and yet act differently while out in the field. But you think that maybe you can be part of the solution and help both sides get along and take the promotion.

Feeling placed in the middle and manipulated. Sometimes by both sides! Trying to stay out of the light of management but they know this. Always testing you to see if you could be "one of the boys" and to see how well you play in their sandbox!

During one meeting, your eyes were truly opened about how they talk about everyone and everything. God, they say woman are bad gossips. Hating their meetings, as they can tear anything about anyone apart. If they really did not like the way you looked or if you did not bow down to them, they went after you with a vengeance. Their favorite sayings were, "F em, fire em" and "It is what it is". Sayings that are still disliked to this day.

They seemed to only remember the bad things that were just normal everyday human occurrences and none of the good that was done. That is, unless the good benefited them and then it was only good for that moment. Nasty and vengeful they were.

A question came up to you about what to do with an employee, who accidentally broke a piece of equipment, as it does happen in the field. You, looking at both sides of the situation state your case and are automatically confronted with "the Boss" saying "Look at you, trying to be fair". Everyone else is just laughing. 'What a bunch of puppets', you thought. Trying to figure a way to put this to stroke their egos you state that there would be repercussions if they carried out the punishment they had in mind. For that punishment far outweighed the crime. You, therefore, do not agree and do not wish to be part of it. Holy crap, the other managers looked at you with their mouths literally hanging open. You with all honesty look at them and wonder what is wrong? You told them that you have a reason, and it should be heard, as it would not reflect well on us or on the department. The boss received a phone call at that moment, and the other managers looked at you, and asked you how you could say no to the boss. "Is that not why we are put in charge?" you ask. Are we not the go-betweens of doing the right things for the department and the employees? Without skipping a beat, the other two numbskulls stated that they never say no, you are supposed to do exactly what the boss wants, be it right or wrong. This goes against your morals. You were then told that you were not playing well in the sandbox and that you needed to be on board with them if you want to do this job. You were reminded that you were no longer a union employee. Wow, after that, you did not always agree, but you did not say anything. You just sat at the meetings and let them go on their rants, and you would help your crews later. You felt like a traitor to your crews. Wondering if you were you now considered one of them?

I remember being so embarrassed at who I was and feeling undeserving. I often said, "This is what I chose, so now I need to deal with it". When it comes to those I was serving, I did as I believed I was supposed to do for both sides. Here I was, trying to make everyone else happy, while being so unhappy in my situation.

Do you ever feel down because you know what is going on is wrong? You are supposed to protect the crews and yet you will be leaving yourself out in the open. You do not wish to be like management and maybe, just maybe, there is a way. You are not sure how it will go but you learned to write things up that you did not agree with in a "as per so and so" manner. You send emails, confirming what you were asked to do for which you are pulled into the office and chastised about. They do not like things in writing and only do phone calls so there is no paper trail.

It makes things tough, you see, after disagreeing with their ways and letting them know about the emails you are writing to yourself, they are leaving you out of situations that you do not wish to be part of. Sure, they are making things tough for you but the crew members are stepping up to help. They see the care put out for them and heard of some of the stances taken, and now without hesitation come in on their time to help with what needs to be done.

It is at this point that you learn to accept the help, which gives you the strength to continue. What you put out is what you receive. It is because of doing the right thing for them that you gained their respect and assistance.

They were the best people anyone could ask for and not only did they rescue others, they helped rescue me.

What we need to understand is that fear can be one huge distraction. Sure, in the fight or flight response it is extremely important. We can take fear and look it in the face. We can take steps to lessen it and move forward. If we allow the fear to grow within us, it just keeps us from stepping out of our comfort zone and never knowing what could truly be. It is those who despite fear act upon their dreams or changes they wish to make who become accomplished.

Chapter 4

Fear Not

"The gem cannot be polished without friction, no man perfected without trials."

- Confucius

Yes, those nuns did make a straight A student out of me but it came at a price. It made me quite paranoid about making any mistakes. Even the good grades came with fear as I was asked numerous times if I was sure of something prior to having the answer accepted. This was all learned in second grade. Sister Philemona, had the belief that you should be perfect in everything and to be confident in your answers. Using the pointer or yardstick was her way of making you so smart. Giving three whacks over the knuckles for any wrong answer on a test. She taught me to not have any type of failure through the tactic of fear! For her, anything less than 100%, was failure. For my father as well. He did not hit me, but he had that look of disappointment. I learned that every action has a consequence, but I really became aware of the negative consequences. Fearing any decisions made became a way of life for me. There could be no mistakes because, with mistakes came punishment. That punishment I learned from her could come from God, my parents or my teachers. Fear of making mistakes, for the ruler would be coming! Even a good consequence at that time came with fear!

I clearly remember a time, standing in front of the class with Mary. We were crying and holding onto each other as we both asked the question, "How could anyone receive not one, but two zeros on a test"? OMG, we asked each other, how was it possible to do worse than a zero. We were only seven and our imaginations were running wild with how bad this was. Berated and hysterical, believing we were going to get the beating of a lifetime. I know I was thinking about how I could not tell my parents nor would I want to. They would be so disappointed in me! She allowed us to stand there in front of the whole class hysterical, for what seemed like forever, prior to telling us that we were the only ones to receive a 100% on our tests that day.

It took me a while, but I have learned not to resent what happened to me throughout my life, because I know that I would not be who I am today without those moments. Allowing myself to have a different perspective on all the happenings of life has helped me grow in ways I never thought I could. I do not hold onto the anger as I once did and I see people differently. It took a long time for me to be able to accept anything below a perfect score. It was not until my children started going to school and seeing them sweat out their grades that I realized that less than perfect should be ok.

I once heard 'the greater the trials and tribulations the greater the reward'. I believe that many of us have had many great trials and tribulations and now it is time for the rewards to come forth. It is time for everyone to take off the masks, the facades and to take down the fences that we built out of defense for ourselves so that we can face life fully without judgments, especially judgments of ourselves! Living life without judgment and with confidence is one of the best rewards.

We are our own worst enemies who need to accept that life is full of lessons and when those lessons are taken and learned, then there is nowhere to go but up! And oh, how good it finally feels to get this!

Fears cost is plenty! It is the one distraction that stops us from ever accomplishing. And that goes for every aspect of our lives. The problem is that we have become so conditioned by fear and we believe it is necessary for us to successfully accomplish life! OK, for the survival instinct of fight or flight, it is. But the sad part is we are not accomplishing, we are existing, and miserably at that. It has become so embedded in us, that it has become part of our every thought and action. We are allowing ourselves to be controlled and manipulated by fear, experiencing the superficial, yet yearning for more. Can we totally get rid of fear? No, I don't believe so, but, we can learn to take it look it in the eye and say WTH, I am going for it. The pros of doing so outweigh the cons of sitting stagnant.

Every hero we have ever heard of or read about was not without fear, they just had an FU attitude and acted despite fear! Fear has caused me to make many mistakes in life. It even ruined my relationship with my children for a while. I had tried to do what I thought would be best, but I feared boundaries.

There were times where I wanted to do what I thought would be best but fear stepped in and stopped me. It robbed me of so much happiness and lost time.

I knew my life was falling apart. Things I refused to accept did not just go away. They built up until they hit me hard and I had no choice but to acknowledge them. Finally, after hearing the whisperings of my coworkers and wanting proof of my husband's extra-curricular activities, I confronted the woman I believed was his girlfriend. She was someone who I supervised at work. It was ironic in that she was sitting with me just hours before I decided to ask her, telling me how she wanted to be just like me and wished she had my life. WOW! Really? No, I did not get upset I felt sorry for her. I tried to explain that she needed to be careful what she wished for. I did ask her and she began to cry. She was so young, twenty years my junior and had those rose-colored glasses on. She only saw my mask. I honestly asked her to see my life as it really was. I even asked her, "If he is so in love with you, why won't he leave me?" Nothing but a blank stare and a promise that she would not take my kids away from me.

You see, I was easily manipulated because of fear and was really beginning to know it. The lies from everyone were so overwhelming. I knew there were lies, but I could not prove it. I tried to bring out the lies for confirmation, through guilt or manipulation. I could not be forward because I feared being wrong! I feared hurting the kids. They feared being hurt by him and they were frightened of him hurting me. And so, it hurt everyone! It became such a vicious cycle.

I had pulled away from everyone and became so damn depressed. Almost ready to accept this as my life. But no more! It was time for me to stand on my own for my children. As I learned at that point, the only person I could count on to change my life was me. I prayed to God that He would help me with this. I did not want to continue to lose myself as well as let my children down. I vowed I would not lose anything more because of it!

Living in fear cost me many things including relationships with the rest of my family for quite some time. I was embarrassed and feared that they would think less of me, as I was always the strong one and had to hold on to that persona. I was easily manipulated and knew it and did not want anyone else to know that. There was an abusive relationship that even had family members believing that I was the one causing all the problems. It was time for me to stand on my own. Yes, I was scared!

Think about what are you afraid of! No, it is not easy, life seems to be fear based and we are a society who accepts running from fear. Fear of the unknown is huge and has so many parameters of 'what if?' What if this, what if that, what if they do not like who I become? Will I like me? Will I be who I am supposed to be?

Take your power and be the Hero. Be your hero! Remember, a hero is not one who does not fear, but, despite fear, pulls on her big girl panties and says enough and pushes through.

Chapter 5

Stop Apologizing

"If you really want to do something you will find a way; if you do not, you will find an excuse."

-Author unknown

You have begun to take notice of your numbness and you are beginning to realize that you are not living up to the potential dreams and wants that you used to have. In fact, you are not even sure who you are anymore. You have lost sight of yourself and do not even know when the last time you saw yourself was. You do not remember your dreams, for they have been pushed so far into the deepest darkest areas of your mind. Yes, you may tell yourself that some dreams are just fairy tales for children, but our dreams are what make us and keep us true to who we are. You should never stop dreaming; the day that you stop dreaming is the day you stop living.

You have stopped living and did not even know it. You have been through many traumas, yes, but the time has come for you to know, it is your decision on how you allow your life to show up. How you live is totally up to you. You can choose to be a victim of life and all that has happened, or you can cowgirl up and get back on that horse and take everything as a lesson to learned. I believe there is something that wants to be taught to us, in all our actions and reactions. All the traumas, successes and failures are because of choices we have or have not made in the past. Making no choice is choosing; it is choosing the victim role. This allows you to believe that you played no part in the situations for which you were put into and lived with. There are times where choices are made for you and for the short term you may need to deal with whatever the situation is, but you can choose to make it short term as you decide how to make your next move. That is making a choice. Not every choice needs to be reactionary and immediate. In fact, a lot of reactionary choices are not always the wisest of choices. You need to decide whether you wish to change the way things are or remain living in the situation that you have chosen.

Are you happy with who you are and how you respond to situations in your life? You are now at your crossroads because your eyes have been opened. The thing about opening your eyes is that you cannot un-see all that was brought into focus. You cannot unlearn all that you have learned. It is like someone telling you not to think about the pink elephant in the room. Too late, you have already put a picture of it in your mind prior to trying to forget about it.

As humans and with the human conditioning, you have learned any change can be extremely difficult and oh so scary. You say to yourself, "Oh my God," and go through all the what ifs. Well let me ask you this, what if you never try? Ask yourself, what is it worth to you and to who you are, to change? What would you, or could you accomplish with this change? And if you stayed in the same crap, what would you lose? Is there anymore of you left to lose? What would the people in your world lose if you were never to be who you were meant to be? Such as your children, who your life revolves around, and they look up to you to teach them.

I believe what scares us most about change is, we believe that it needs to be completely painful and full of heartache. Your knowledge of the state of mind you are in is one of the biggest steps and one of the biggest obstacles to changing. It is like an addict finally admitting to having a problem. You now see, but do you have the acceptance of how your life really is without the masks? Are you feeling all your emotions reeling inside? Like a whirlpool that was so wide but now you are finally nearing the funnel and it is time, scary because you are nearing the drain. What do you do? You can choose to continue to place your emotions into that special junk room you built in your mind. Something you have done so often as to not deal with them. Just understand, pent up emotions build with enormous strength, sending cracks through the mortar of your wall. Those cracks will extend and weaken your wall of defense, until you are left with nothing to hold them in. As they come out in a flood, they become overwhelming and paralyzing. How are you supposed to deal with all at once, what you have always put aside? Self-loathing and unhappiness can come flooding in.

I knew my life was falling apart. Things I refused to accept did not just go away. They built up until they hit me hard and I had no choice but to acknowledge them. I always felt I could not change things until I had concrete proof in my hands to serve on a silver platter. That meant for me the murmurings of everyone at work, who talked amongst themselves but said nothing to me. They would all become silent and or change the subject when I came around. They were afraid of telling me anything. I always say a wife knows, and deep down I knew, but after being told by some that I was imagining things or was just afraid, I feared being wrong. What would I do if I confronted him and did the unthinkable of throwing him out and I was wrong? Always looking at the judgment and worried what the others may think. Hell, our marriage really sucked, but as I stated earlier, for better or worse and I got worse. If only I could finally have proof of my husband's extra-curricular activities.

I think what really woke me up was the fact that Glenn's girlfriend honestly believed that *she* would let me keep my children. *OMG REALLY? TRIGGER!* That was my biggest reason for wanting a life change. It took a few moments, but then it hit me, I realized then and there that I was looking at who I was when I began dating him! It was at this point that I knew I would not get through to her and that I needed to do what is right for me! I did ask her to please help me get him out of my house and told her that I wished them both the best of luck. And with that went home.

How do you change all that is wrong? You must come to realize that all of life is not your fault. You are not to blame for things not going right in someone's life other than your own. Each person is responsible for his or her own actions and that includes their actions upon others. The only other person, besides yourself, for whom you are responsible is the children you bring into this world and even that is temporary. For they grow with your guidance and hopefully learn from you how to be strong and reliable and confident in all that they do! They do watch and learn. You are their first teacher and for that you must be careful in what is taught to them.

If our children see us as the peacekeepers who become apology ridden it can cause them to see us as weak or see weakness as how you are supposed to be and take on your actions. They have learned that apologies are for forgiveness of something. They see your insecurities, it is time to break the cycle and show them how to be strong and stand up for your beliefs, instead of showing them how to take on the same actions that you have lived. Time to teach through the actions of strength.

Ask yourself, are you always wrong? After all, you do apologize for having feelings; you apologize for apologizing. Your constant apologies cause fear, and fear allows manipulation and causes you to spiral into insecurities.

We all need to learn that throughout our lives we are not going to please all the people we may encounter. We may also find that we may not even please the same people on a consistent basis.

Did you know that over apologizing can become self-destructive? What is meant to dissolve hostile situations and to encourage forgiveness can cause self-destruction if used improperly. Using apologies on a reactive basis for things that are not even within your control gives an appearance of lack of confidence, competence, and professional judgment. After hearing it from yourself for so long your mind even begins to believe it too. Why else would you say it so much if it was not true. Therefore, it brings others to doubt your abilities especially as a leader. We tend to apologize for things we are insecure about. Even though we know they are not our fault, we still feel badly about the incidents and by over apologizing consistently we instill a belief in ourselves and others that we deserve the blame of doubt. We lose confidence in ourselves.

How do we stop? Begin by saying thank you! When someone does the dishes for us, do not immediately go into the mode of "I should have", I did not accomplish, no self-flagellating instead, just say thank you! Stop taking blame for things that are not your fault.

Withholding an apology can be empowering. Take a breath, pause and say thank you instead.

Chapter 6

Happiness Comes from Within

Happiness is the one thing that everyone is always looking for. Where do you find it? Can you buy it? Can someone give it to you? You search high and low, is it on the other side of the fence where the grass is greener? What is it that you are looking for? Fill in the blank, I will be happy when _____. Look and see what it is you are looking for. Does it involve external seeking?

As a person brought up in today's society, you are taught that happiness comes from the material goods you obtain throughout your life. Always reaching higher and higher for that is what we believe as a society brings happiness. The more it costs the better you will feel and the happier you will be.

I had an EMT from another unit one day, while on a standby, tell me that he and his wife met a couple while at a school outing with their kids. This couple owned a Lexus. He explained that they thought this would be a nice couple to get to know basically based on the luxury car. He was so dismayed when he found out they were regular people who did not have a home that would be in Better Homes magazine. This, I must say, was the same person who did not have children over his house often as it would mean having a mess. I felt sorry for his children.

Always wearing your mask of perfection and having your labels. But when have you been truly happy? As an EMT, saving others is your happiness, when you help someone it feels good, it is that feeling which brings an inner peace to you. You see, when you were younger, happiness was sought through your parents. Seeing them happy with your actions is what brought you your happiness. So, as an adult, what brings you your happiness?

I believe that it is our ego way of thinking which has brought us to the external searching for happiness. It is the labels and categories and always trying to be better than the Jones'. When we are not happy with ourselves, we believe that obtaining that illustrious trophy of a big house, money or job is what will bring us the happiness we deserve. There are people who have reached this success and who have not found happiness. One reason is that they then become fearful of losing it. What do they do? They hold onto it tightly in a miserly way, never enjoying it or allowing others in to enjoy it with them. We always hear that happiness lies within. Well then how the heck do we find it?

One of the first things to do is to take yourself away from negative people. Hanging around with the negative people can be so draining. Constantly hearing how nothing in life is good, and always having the victim mentality. Gossiping about those who seem happy. They are always judging others, their looks, their actions, what they have or don't have. Being in a group of people can bring you to a like-minded way of thinking. If you keep thinking 'poor me', well then that is the standard you are going to keep setting yourself up to live by. Always the victim, never having anything of worth. By putting yourself into a more positive group of people, you can find that life is more pleasurable. Who knows, you may even find that you have more than you thought you did!

Another way to rid yourself of negative speak is to change your story. How about telling yourself only positive things. Make it a challenge; you know you like challenges. Every time you hear yourself saying something in a negative way, change it to a positive. Do not use statements such as I can't, instead, say I can. Do not wait for things to get better on their own, start now taking one step at a time. Even if you cannot climb that mountain in one day, so what! Each step closer is still a step. This is how affirmations work. Stating the positive over and over until your brain is hearing it so many times that it is now believing it to be the truth. With that comes a confidence and a belief in yourself. Affirmations will not work if one really doubts that they are deserving or worthy of something. Begin with the little obvious things, such as 'you are good'. You are smart. I let only positive in and positive out. Move on to 'I am happy'. I deserve. And just keep on telling yourself, because it is true. Change your perception. At the end of the book, there is a free download of affirmations to help you get started.

Take challenges as growth. I always used to hear from my father, "What doesn't kill you, only makes you stronger." I now see that as truth. You see you do not realize that you have faced so many challenges already in your life. Think about this, you have made it through each one, even when you believed you never would. How cool is that? You do not realize that as hard as it may have been, you have learned and you grew from every experience you had. Change your perception and you change your story. Instead of being the victim, be the one who kicked butt! Yeah, I lived through that ordeal, I survived and look at me now getting stronger!

Speaking of kicking butt, if you were to always be in the warrior mode of kicking butt, that would hold you in the drama mode of negative. It is wise to pick and choose your battles. Ask yourself if something is really that important. Will it affect you at the end of today, tomorrow or next year? Most of our fights with partners, children or friends are so insignificant that we cannot even remember what they were about. Most times it is a fight over control and the need to be right. We do not need to always be right, we are human and we are expected to be wrong at times. It does not make you less than anyone else.

We all learn by doing. Mozart, even as gifted as he was, had to practice and make mistakes. But I bet he just kept going and no one noticed or cared!

Learn to live in the now. Remember, the past is done and cannot be changed. What can be changed is your perception of it and how you can release your attachment to it. We tend at times to hold onto the past so tightly that we never even see what we have now. Every time you say, "Do you know what he did to me?" It only brings you right back to where you were, as if it is still going on. It keeps you in the perpetual victim mode, and keeps you angry, especially if they have moved on. It all becomes a what about me thing. Well, what about you? Choose to move forward by releasing the pain. Acknowledge it is there and let it go.

One way of releasing your emotions is by writing. It does not have to be legible, or grammatically correct, it is just for you. Just get out a pen/pencil and paper and start writing. You can start by writing, "I do not know how to begin to say what I want to say about how I feel about what so and so did but…" Do not worry, just get it out. When you have written a few lines, you will begin to write without thinking about writing. Your feelings will naturally start coming out. Let them. Be blunt, be honest. You will find that you will begin to lighten up when you are nearing the finish. That is good. You can end it with, "I no longer wish to hold onto any of these feelings as they do not serve me in any positive way. I release them." With that, tear the paper into a million pieces, or crumple it up tightly and throw it away. Some people like to burn it. Take it outside and in a fireproof container light the paper and let it burn until it is nothing but ashes.

Let go of what you allowed or did not allow by forgiving yourself. Realize that everyone has a story and that you are not the only one who is afraid. You did the best you could, with what you had and what you knew. Remember the fact that you are only human and are expected to make mistakes. We all do. Think of all that it has taught you. Think of all that you can pass onto others. But know, if others are not ready to hear it or learn from your experience, just as you were not learning from someone else's, they will not take your advice. You need to accept that and move on. Trying to control someone does not make anyone happy, either you or them. It brings annoyance and frustration.

Boundaries are helpful and can keep you happy. What is a boundary? A boundary is a metaphorical fence that you build and let people know not to cross over. It allows people to know what you will and will not accept for yourself and for others. It sets up that respect line. You need to give respect to get respect. I am sure you have heard that, but that includes for yourself! Give yourself respect if you expect others to give it to you. Boundaries allow you to have love for yourself that you do deserve. We are all deserving of boundaries and no one is made to be walked on by another. No matter who you are or where you were brought up. Boundaries create happiness in you.

You will find that there are people who do not believe in having boundaries put upon them, but, they will have boundaries that they do not wish for you to cross. These are usually the ones who manipulate and twist situations to their favor. They may try other ways to go around your boundaries, pulling on your guilt strings and playing the victim role very well. When I made my changes, it threw people off their game.

Always remember that no one is perfect. Looking for perfection, in yourself, in others or in the things you or they do, only leads to undue stress. Learn when to stop and accept 'good enough'.

When doing any self-help, do not expect any immediate changes. It takes time to change and it is stated that for a person to change their habit it can take two to eight months to accomplish. Look at each day for the change is happening.

Take challenges and break them into doable steps. Each day complete one small step and before you know it you are done.

Chapter 7

Change Your Story, Change Your Life

"Hypnosis has been referred to as a belief in fantasy. It's a trance like state and not some weird thing. We go in and out of trances every day. Think of hypnosis as a perceptual adjustment."

-Carol Denicker, NY Hypnosis Training Center

What made the most changes for me? Hypnosis did. I must admit, I do not like the word hypnosis because of all the negative connotations that come along with it. I can remember seeing it performed in movies and on TV. I can recall the stage hypnotists who could make you cluck like a chicken or do things in public that you would normally be embarrassed to do. These representations have brought a bad rap to hypnosis. All these myths, brought through the ages give hypnosis a perceived definition of a person being controlled, and total surrender of self, and morals to the hypnotist.

I personally thought of hypnosis as 'mind control' based on the old black and white TV shows that I saw when I was younger. I remember hearing about hypnosis from someone in a group that I went to for self-help. There was no way I was ever going to even think of doing that! That said, how do I expect you to believe what I say about it? I will just tell you what I know in my heart now and leave it up to you!

Even though I went to some group sessions prior to a one on one, I still had that belief of being safer in a group setting than with a one on one. I realize now, I was just more afraid of finding things out about myself that I did not want to know, or want others to know. I was someone who needed to remain in control and was afraid of losing that part of myself, even for a moment. Nothing can be further from the truth. It was my mentor and teacher, Carol Denicker, who showed me the reality of hypnosis. She is so good and passionate about her teaching that she has a school in Long Island, New York that is the first State Certified School for hypnosis. She made me realize that hypnosis is a great tool. I found that it allowed my body to relax as if sedated and yet my mind was super aware! I remember thinking that I may start to drool, which should have awoken me immediately, but I thought, oh well, what the heck. I am too comfortable. If I wanted to, I could have chosen to end the session right then and there and walk out. Trust me, I was so comfortable and did not want to stop! It is because of her that I am a hypnotist today and have a great tool for helping people in their process.

Hypnosis works on the subconscious part of your mind. The part of the mind that you do not think about. It is a part of your mind that allows the automatic reactions for the situations you may be in.

Hypnosis integrated with visualization, affirmations and/ or just plain old meditation can help to do wonders for you and take years off your journey. We are always on that journey to grow, or I believe we should be always trying to improve ourselves. Hypnosis, be it with a hypnotist or self-hypnosis is such a wonderful quickener for those who are trying to make changes.

You see the mind is an amazing thing. We really do not understand so much about its untapped potential but one of the most amazing things to me is that it is like a computer with infinite storage space. It remembers every little action or reaction, from every aspect of your life. It does not always know the "real" from the imagined. In that, in a session that is integrated with visualizations, you can make your mind know that this is a reality for you that you are expecting to happen. It can also believe that you do not want an action anymore and therefore will make the changes. It is important to know that you can talk yourself out of anything. Holding a belief makes it a reality to the mind!

I have often heard that we are part of a reality and still do not understand that to the fullest. I know that the more I learn, the more I question with the realization that I do not know much. I believe that every person has a different reality and truth which holds true for them. It is similar to how it is sometimes said, life is like 'The Matrix'. It is up to us to take the red or blue pill. I now understand for me that the red and blue pills are perspectives. It is what we choose in our wants needs and our *reality*. We can go along with society and stay where we are or we can become individuals who blaze that trail.

Take the example of two children growing up in the same family. Basically, you have the same parameters for both children. They are in a family of two parents who are drunkards and abusive to each other. They neglect their children the same.

But you can have from the same environment, one child who grows up to be successful in everything he does in life. He sees everything as an experience of life and learns what he does not wish to be or accept. Yet, the other child will see things in a victim role mentality, always wondering what he did to deserve all this. What is the difference between the children? Their perspective.

How we perceive life and its situations can make or break us. I remember a time when I would become upset over someone trying to control my every move. Now, I realize, it is my choice whether I allow this person to do such a thing. I can take charge of my life and its actions, or allow and just be in the constant barrage of the victim mentality. It was hypnosis that allowed me to have a perceptual adjustment enough, to now *believe*, that it was time to pull up my big girl panties. I always knew I *had* to do that, but the *belief that I could* was not there.

Hypnosis allows you to become focused and work on a specific goal. Even though other thoughts may come up, you can acknowledge that thought and have it move on. There are times though, that the thought comes in as a reason that you were blocking yourself from accomplishing a goal or belief. This thought can be adjusted from affecting you negatively at that moment.

Some wonder whether hypnosis and the thoughts or visualizations are real or imagined. Everyone has their differing beliefs on that and I believe it to be ok to have either thought. Some people may have both.

Every journey that one takes should be a private journey of self. It should not be looked at for acceptance from all those around you, to decide what does or does not work for you. There are so many who believe hypnosis to be a mind controlling tool and it will be impossible to change their mind unless they experience it for themselves.

No one in life can *make* you do anything that you do not wish to do! Those people that you see on stage with a hypnotist who makes them cluck like chickens, actually do want to be part of the show, running around clucking like chickens. If you pay close attention, you will see that the hypnotist picks who he/she knows will be easily suggestible. In other words, the hypnotist is looking for the one who would allow and follow the suggestions given.

There are also people who are in the camp of believing that they can never be hypnotized, even if they wanted to. Some people are truly into total control and as I said before, it cannot happen without you allowing it to happen. That does not mean that it can never happen for them, it just means that they need to find someone that they trust and build a rapport with. Trust is one of the biggest, most important factors when doing hypnosis.

To come to trust your hypnotist, have a rapport with them, you should have a first session that is extended in time for the both of you to get to know each other, what you are looking for and what you are and are not comfortable with. It should flow, and you should be calm. Sure, a little nervousness is expected the first time, but you know the difference between butterflies and downright 'get out of Dodge' feeling. What is the worst that can happen? Is that you will not have a hypnotic experience and that the hypnotist will leave you with a bad taste in your mouth about all hypnotists.

Just as in every profession, there are good and bad or just mediocre. I remember when a client who claimed to be the biggest skeptic came in for a session. She was an EMT friend who stated that she did not think she could be hypnotized and wanted to prove to everyone in the field that this was a waste of time. We wanted to pick a topic that she wished to work on. She chose her fear of riding her horse, as she lost all confidence in that and had recently became fearful. Even though she was not an avid rider like the rest of her family, she would get on a horse and just walk for hours. She was a little defensive initially. Stating, "I am one of those who you can't make do anything!" I agreed with her, and asked her why she came. I think the wind blew out of her sails as she was ready with a defense and did not get to use it. We spoke for a while and she stated she was ready to try. We did a short trance relaxation for her to became comfortable. She almost seemed disappointed and asked if she was truly in hypnosis, because she heard every sound that happened in the room. She felt she was thinking her own thoughts and could ignore me if she wanted to. Always feeling in control and capable of accepting or not accepting what was being said.

I had not heard anything from her for a few months, as we worked different sectors of the five boroughs, but then, she called to say, "I wanted to not be so scared and learn how to ride without fear. She explained that she had become afraid of riding her horse and any other horse. She called to tell me that immediately after our session, she ran to the barn and signed up for the horse shows (competitions) which were beginning in less than two weeks. Everyone at the barn was cheering her on. She had never taken a lesson and ridden properly, she did not even trot or lope. There for so many years, she did all the ground work but never rode. It was a show barn too! Guess what? She took Grand Champion for the season!

She explained that during the session, she was told to visualize herself riding her horse and couldn't. She pictured a horse of a different color. She tried not to think anything of it. Wouldn't you know the first day of lessons and as she was riding, she looked down and saw what she visualized in our session. At the end of the show season, she stated, "I took *my* horse out, saddled her up and it was the proudest moment for me in a long time". She did everything I asked, we loped, trotted, switched leads everything! There were no trees, electric fences, no bucking or refusals! I even let the kids watch!"

Hypnosis in general works. And allows you to adjust the way your subconscious perceives things. It can change your story. It is as simple sometimes as changing your story, as told with this client Rob.

Rob was a virtuoso violinist in an orchestra that played in NYC. He came for a session as he was tired of his anxiety routine prior to any performance. He would become nauseous and throw up prior to going onstage. He did go for therapy for a while for this issue and found that he could not find the reason why. It was quite a few months and the issue was still there. He came in frustrated and explained the story of what happened prior to every performance. After going into a trance-state he was given the suggestions of the positive changes he wished to achieve, to change the storyline of what happens prior to his performances.

I received a phone call approximately one week later. It was Rob, who was astounded that he was fine prior to his first performance after the session. He asked for the magic trick and all that could be said was, "We just changed your story. During the session, we worked on what story you wanted to partake in and adjusted your perception. Now that became the story your subconscious mind understood to be what happens prior to and during any performance."

Remember, the analogy of the mind being like a computer. It remembers every reaction you have had, to every action you have faced. It remembers what worked for you in the past and keeps it in files of 'great reactions to have', 'saved your hide' or something like that. So, any time you have a trigger that seems similar, that becomes your automatic reaction.

One of the problems of holding onto the same reaction for so long is that you can outgrow your reactions What worked for you when you were seven and just learning about life, may not be right for you now. But just as you learned that we hold onto our labels, our mind keeps our responses. So, here we have a belief that is outdated and doing us no good. Time to adjust your thinking, your story, your perception. I know that it sounds so difficult. But it really is not. There is not much to tell you about the magical part of the hypnosis, just that it does change the way you react to things.

For any habit to change it is said that it takes an average of two to eight months of working on it. That means a process of changing our minds, adjusting our perception. While doing it on your own it may become difficult while having a bad day. It can become an obstacle. We can then find that while it went well for a week we may fall back into our old routine. It is like having to remember to take our vitamins every day, twice a day. There are times we remember but then forget. Life gets in the way. Yes, it is possible but it just means working harder. That is where with hypnosis I learned instead of working harder, I can work smarter. It does not mean that I do no work, of course. I must want the changes that I am looking for, but it helps the mind to integrate the process into our everyday living starting right away.

Chapter 8

Taking A Shortcut

I was talking with Brian Katcher, an old coworker from my paramedic days and asked him the question, "If I Am So Strong, Why Do I Feel So Weak"? His statement was immediate. It was to me, something that struck a chord as to how I was perpetuating in my mind the issue of being the fixer of everyone else and not myself. He stated, "Because like many of us, your training was to hide your humanity for the benefit of those around you. To show strength and hide weakness, lest it show through to those who needed us to be a wall. We, in this job, are all horribly broken. Our strength is our internal weakness. Our weakness is our outward strength".

I see that these problems of experiencing guilt for saying no, the feeling of being taken advantage of, the inability of showing any weakness, can become compounded with the job that you have chosen. Being so compelled to help everyone and be of value to them. To do the job as rescuer, fixer and healer of everyone around you, you have learned all too well, how to only show the strength that you have. And so, what started out as being a good thing for those around you, has become in your mind, for you, a weakness. You have become so used to the role of being that wall that your strength in helping others has become your weakness. There is good news though, it does not have to remain that way.

Knowing this is the start of fixing it. It is through the knowledge of the what and the why you are doing what you do, that you can make the changes you need. You can become strong for you and be happy doing it. How is this done? It begins by letting go. Letting go of living the lies which you have put into place. All those masks that you made from the fear of being judged, or from the embarrassment of not being who you believe you are expected to be. It is time to live your truth, the truth of who you are. You are a person who born with the same rights as everyone born into this world. Not to be less than, but to be your fullest in everything you do or dream of. You deserve to dream and to be happy. You were taught and lived by your labels and your training from the moment you came to be. You can still do that but with one difference. Doing what is right for you. When you do for you and regain your strength, it is amazing how it positively affects those around you. Your strength, through the acceptance of your weaknesses, brings peace and with that peace comes the confidence and happiness that you long for.

Let me explain, I had been in your shoes at one time and thought that I would never find peace or happiness again. Feeling so incapable and unhappy, just functioning. My marriage was done. It was done for a long time. I was not happy and had a difficult time trying to remember any happiness. There were so many lies. I questioned what was real and what wasn't. I could not tell anymore if I just pretended the whole thing. It was after the validation and proof of my husband's girlfriend that I knew I needed to do something, as I was allowing these situations to remain. Now that my eyes were open, the ball was in my court.

So, scary, as I felt that I would never find love or happiness. No one would want me. Hell, if my own husband didn't want me, why would anyone else? My insecurities were huge. I only had my job which gave me solace, in the helping of others. Everything else seemed a chore. I kept busy, that kept my mind not thinking. Feeling pulled in so many directions, there was an order of protection brought against Glenn and he lost all rights for quite some time with our kids. Now, I was really all alone. No family to help me, and my friends lived too far away.

Going to court for the order, I had the judge blame me for all the things going on. He was thanking Glenn for being a fine father and an upstanding person. He believed that I, being the scorned woman, was lying about everything. Really? My lawyer, the first one, said nothing and was almost crying after that court session. How was I to make changes when everyone is against me? My lawyer was afraid of this judge and not doing anything! Who was I to think I could ever find happiness. I took the steps and was falling deeper into the pit. I was told I was swaying my children. They knew nothing about what was going on in our private life. My son even thanked me one day for throwing him out! If I told them that, they would swear even more that I was swaying them. Hell, I was being blamed for it anyway. Here I was asking for help and I felt no one was helping. I was being told, I was the problem! The problem that had to pay for forensic therapy for him and the kids, even though I was not allowed to be part of the sessions. I was told by the therapist that I was not the problem in this matter! Ok, so then why am I being blamed and why can't you tell the judge. In which she replied, "Not yet all in due time". She is not due to report to the court for a few months. Really? And why do I have to pay for his issues. He would walk out of court smiling and he and his lawyer would both have things to say within earshot. I wanted to quit. Being strong was for the birds, I thought.

I could have taken the low road and have done what his lawyer and the judge wanted me to do and that was to concede and give up everything. I was now angry, I needed to feel the fire beneath me. What I found was that my conceding and allowing only brought more of the same in. I fired my lawyer and hired a new one. Stood my ground and put myself into the mode of fighting for myself. I needed a newer, better version of me. I was so scared and was not totally convinced I could do this, but I had to so that I could break this cycle, not just for my children, but for me. One of my biggest issues was the fact that I never had anything against him. There was no paper trail, no people to help me because I had always kept things hidden. I hid because of my fear of judgment and embarrassment. All this running from judgment caused me to be judged. Embarrassed because I felt less than what I thought I should be. I allowed myself to be tucked away in the corner. Glenn did not want me growing in any way, because he felt, I would be better than him and he could not stand that. He liked having the upper hand. He did not have to be abusive in a physical way, to hold me back, because he used my own emotions and beliefs against me. The emotional abuse which I allowed. It caused me to hide myself and believe myself to be less than anyone else. It is also much harder to prove as the scars are not always visible.

"If someone can change your mind, he has won you over without raising his hand against you. This is the future of warfare."
-Bangambiki Habyarimana, *Pearls of Eternity*

Once I took the stance and pulled on my big girl panties, things went into a motion immediately for the positive. My new lawyer came out of chambers one day and told me how I was being so screwed over. He could not believe what went on before, but he promised me he would help. I was ecstatic but still a little apprehensive. I did begin to feel as if the light was beginning to show. It was not long after that the truth came out. The judge, who wanted to hold me in contempt on the first day, well, he sent my new lawyer out to apologize to me. Wanting me to be told that he could not come out into the court room, as he would not be able to hold his temper back from my soon to be ex. REALLY? I was upset as I had to endure his BS in the courts every month, sometimes two and three times a month, for over a year. But, the truth was finally revealed and that is all I wanted.

The point of this is please understand, things happen because you allow them to. We allow this through our choice or lack thereof. It takes reflection and looking inside, which is something most of us fear doing. Especially, the first time. We do not want to believe ourselves to be less than perfect.

We always feel the need to be part of the whole to feel as if we are part of something. I believe, that is where we go wrong. In doing so, we allow ourselves to be run by others or the thoughts of what we think the others want us to be and to do. We do this without even thinking about what is going on, and often, we believe ourselves to be not worthy.

Perfection is what we all strive for, but that is a goal that will never be reached. It will never be reached, because we are human and therefore, we will make mistakes. Once we accept this, so many of the trivial things in our life just won't matter anymore. It is when we put on the masks and live the lies that we do not obtain what it is we are truly seeking. We attract what we believe and that can be all that is not good. For when we doubt ourselves and have negative thoughts of being unworthy, that will be what we receive.

Belief in yourself can be the most difficult thing to obtain. I say, believe in yourself for you already have come such a long way. Your eyes have been opened and you are regaining your strength. Look at and be proud of how you have begun to find the fire for yourself. It is sad that it took so much misery, but now is the time to take that misery as a lesson of growth and forgive yourself. Do not hold yourself to 'would have, should have, could have', because that is when we stay stuck in the muck of misery. When you can forgive yourself, it is wonderful how you can forgive others as well. Remember, forgiveness and letting go does not mean forgetting and allowing. You are not giving up. It means that you are not holding onto the attachment from people, their outcomes or situations. You and then see the lessons in the actions taken or not taken. You can and will find then, the energy to put into your hopes and dreams. This energy put in, without the desperate stress of it needing only one specific outcome, can be freeing and inspiring for endless possibilities.

There is deep down a belief that you do have in you, for you. If it were not there, you would not be searching for answers. Know that you have begun your journey.

Standing up for yourself, no matter how small you may believe yourself to be, is a start. Creation of boundaries is healthy for you, as it gives you a love and a respect for yourself, as well those around you. As for the haters, just know that the people who are truly your friends will understand your boundaries and work with you. You are just as deserving as anyone else, for we are all born with the same rights of Happiness, Love, Compassion and Respect.

What I would really want to say to my former self while going through her situation is; "I don't know if you realize that it took great strength to move forward while in the face of your fear of being judged. I know that you are scared now that you are on your own, but you are also feeling that sense of freedom you have. It does take some getting used to. It is not the absence of fear that allows people to grow it is their actions, despite their fear. You will continue to have the distractions of fear, especially of those around you, but you will find that each day it has less and less of a hold on you. And now that your eyes are open, you will notice it more easily and not allow it to take hold of you. You need to remember that going back into your fear and allowing it to spiral down will only bring you back to where you were. Always hold onto the growth that you have each day. No matter how trivial you believe it to be. Live for the moment and not in the future or in the past. The past is done, the future is affected by what you do today. So, living each day and appreciating what is in front of you will bring wondrous things".

Happiness is within each one of us. It is not in the quantity of friends you have, but in the quality of your friends. No one can make you happy but you. Any partner in life should be just that, a partner who is there to grow with you, you cheer each other on in your joint adventures as well as your individualized ones. A partner does not think about what are you going to do for me, but of what do I have for you to help you grow and you lovingly and happily accept it. You have found happiness in the simple things and have learned to love yourself. You have created boundaries that are healthy for you and those around you.

The biggest steps that anyone can take, are asking for help, saying 'Thank you' instead of 'I am sorry' and having appreciation for someone wanting to do something for them.

Remember, no one is perfect and anyone who leads you to believe that they are, needs to be let go of. Keeping drama in your life will only bring you drama. Surround yourself with positive people. If you need to be with negative people, shorten your time with them and keep your boundaries. If you are called nasty names because you are doing what is right for you, take it and wear it as a badge with pride. Be assertive and hold your boundaries. Realize that these actions are a sign of weakness and insecurity in the person saying this. Try not to judge them, but do not give in to them. Everyone has a story and if we take the high road of respect, maybe it will rub off on them. If not, hold your head high and walk away.

If you take anything away from this book, just always remember that in life, you are going to find that you cannot please everyone. Nor should you have to. There are going to be those haters who you thought were your friends. I believe that they, even if not on a conscious level, do not want to see growth in you. This can hold true even more so if they are unhappy. Your growth in your happiness can create in them self-reflection and judgment.

There are all kinds of people in this world and I thank God for that. It would be so boring if we were all the same. We can find happiness in all walks of life. I believe, contrary to many of my family members, you do not need to have college degrees, or be CEOs, to lead a productive life. It is not for everyone. My son for example, went on to a prestigious school to become a nuclear engineer, only to move onto finance and now is working his own business in a trade working with horses! Kudos to him for breaking conformity and being happy in what he is doing! That is what makes a person great inside and out. He was always pegged as the smart one, who would make all the plans of the world, by some and felt the need to live out that label for quite some time, especially after the death of his father. He needed to prove that he could achieve something so difficult because that is what was expected of him, he thought. Especially expected of himself. But he was not happy in the least. I am happy that he found his strength and confidence at such a young age to step into what he loves, his passion. Too many of us grow old in our labels and it becomes more difficult for us to let go of who we believe we should be. If you accomplish anything in this life, it should be to teach your children to experience everything. Leading by example is the best way. Too many of us become stagnant in our labels of what a perfect person should be. Be that child that sings, no matter how out of tune it may sound and dance like no one is watching.

What I hope you have gained from this book is that there is hope. That no one is incapable of obtaining their goal. The biggest thing is to believe in yourself even if for a millisecond and get that fire going. It may start out as an ember but that ember can burst into the biggest fire there ever was!

Everything is so doable for someone who is trying to gain their confidence in any area of their life. The biggest trick is that you must want it. And trust me, there are times where even the most confident person in the world needs a little boost. Feeling vulnerable or having the need for assistance is far from negative.

There are people already growing and learning about themselves who come for hypnosis. They have become aware of actions/traits or habits. They come to adjust their perception and quicken the time spent trying to obtain their goal and the results can be great. Hypnosis helps with your connection to the you just waiting to come out!

It is important to understand that hypnosis is not sleep but a meditative state, a state of relaxation in which the mind becomes more aware and clear, more focused and capable of reasoning. There is no loss of control, no loss of consciousness, no surrender of will. One client asked their hypnotist, "What if something were to happen to you while I am under hypnosis?" The hypnotist replied, "Open your eyes and call 911." This is possible because you are always in control and can come out of hypnosis whenever you wish. You are inducing yourself with my guidance, therefore always in control and capable.

Hypnosis promotes wanted life changes. It helps to create those changes on the behavioral, emotional and physical levels. It is a scientifically proven technique and its true purpose is to help you gain more control over your behavioral, emotional and physical well-being. You do not need to be a relaxed person, just willing to allow me to guide you through the process. Hypnosis is truly a deep form of meditation that allows you to connect with the real you hiding inside.

Build a rapport with your hypnotist and be comfortable with what you are doing, as trust is important. Many are creating programs, and hypnosis is being done on a virtual forum either on the computer, or the phone, or both. This may not work for everyone, but it works for many.

I Believe

By Eleanor J Miller

I believe in a world so natural and free
I believe in the love of you and me
Maybe if we just take the chance
The love within us would make us dance
We each have a part to play
And with true love
Nothing is needed to say
If we would all just be real
No masks of fakes
Nothing would be hidden
There would be no mistakes
Just lessons learned
No fear of retaliation
Life would be
One sweet education
Remember it just takes one leap
Have faith in yourself
All it can do is help

Acknowledgements

I have been told for the longest time by so many that I should write a book. I thought about it and then let it go. This went on for quite a while. Last year after life events caused me to change my lifestyle tremendously, I was hearing it from people again. I would ask them, what kind of book? They were not sure but it had to do with what I have learned. I laughed, because what have I learned that no one else knows about?

Moving upstate and having quiet reflection, I began to feel for myself that I needed to write, as clients would ask if I have a book. So many people asking can't be a coincidence. And so, I did. I began writing about my lessons and of the things I went through. I felt there was so much to be said but, was unsure if I was worthy of doing such a thing. I asked for Divine guidance and was lead to Angela Lauria. After speaking with her I felt like she was the one person I needed to guide me in the writing of this book, which I did not know would be *this* book!

Angela, your only true *job* was to guide me in the writing of this book. You have done so much more than that. Your process has challenged me on so many levels and for that I am extremely grateful. I remember our first conversation and my feeling how positive you were, about me being capable of what I did not even know I could do. Thank you for not allowing me to be small, and for standing your ground. I look forward to working together again soon!

I must say, it was a culmination of all my life's experiences both big and small that brought me to where I am at this moment. With that said, I would like to thank all the people who had some of the greatest influences in my life. People like:

My parents. Although mom and Dad have not been here on the Earthly plane for thirty years now, much of who I am now is because of them.

My children, to whom the biggest part of my heart belongs. I have learned so much from you both. You have taught me priorities, and the art of picking and choosing battles. Other lessons learned were Winners clean up, Kiddy scissors suck at cutting hair and Not every lightning bug is a lightning bug. I know that it has not been an easy road, but thank you for choosing me. Even though we may be apart in distance, thoughts of both of you will always tickle my heart! I know I can still be corny and embarrassing!

My bestie friend and sister since forever, Julie! You always championed for me and understood me even when I did not understand myself. You are the one who gave me courage when I did not have the courage to speak to anyone! Thank you for helping me with life! You always were my safe space.

Douglas and Amanda, for your amazing generosity in backing my project.

Chrissy and Keith, for giving me the opportunity to make these amazing life changes.

Cristal my soul sister who has allowed me to express all my concerns, wants and dreams and with so much passion!

Christine, who never thinks anything I say is crazy! I am still amazed at how simple and easy, yet so strong and true, your faith is.

My clients, who have helped me to grow in assisting others. For I grow too, each and every time we come together for a phone session or face-to-face. Thank you for your trust and for allowing yourself to be, at times, vulnerable. Seeing the growth in you is what keeps me so passionate about what we do together. Because of you, this will never be a job, but a life calling!

To the Morgan James Publishing team: Special thanks to David Hancock, CEO & Founder for believing in me and my message. To my Author Relations Manager, Tiffany Gibson, thanks for making the process seamless and easy. Many more thanks to everyone else, but especially Jim Howard, Bethany Marshall, and Nickcole Watkins.

Last but certainly not least, I would like to thank the ones who are always understanding and offer unconditional love on a consistent basis, my three dogs, Smokey, Mikey and Catori. You have listened to me and my ideas and tolerated my hours of endless thinking and writing for this book and the program. (Yes, like the parents of most fur babies, I do talk to them and run ideas past them). You always know when to tell me to take a break, especially at 3pm and dinner time.

About the Author

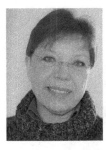 Eleanor is a Reiki Master, Interfaith Minister, a Certified Consulting Hypnotist and is currently obtaining her NLP certification. She believes that everyone has the right to become the authority of his or her own life. She has made it her life's work to help others find their strength and wants to share this message everywhere for everyone to know!

Eleanor lives in New York and has traded in the sirens and traffic of NYC for the coyotes, snakes and other animals that go bump in the night of rural Sharon Springs. Keeping her and her three dogs constantly on their toes.

For more on what Eleanor does, go to:
Website: www.thewondersofyou.com
Email: thewondersofyoullc@gmail.com

Thank You

I would like to take the time to thank you for reading my book. I hope you enjoyed reading it as much as I enjoyed writing it. It is my intention for you to understand that you are not alone, and yes, there can be a happy ending filled with dreams and blue sunny skies. My vision in writing this book has always been that it would serve you in your journey, as you are at one of the crossroads of your life. In saying this, I would like to help you as you begin the next part of your journey.

Please go to www.thewondersofyou.com to receive your daily affirmations. A 3 step Self-Hypnosis tutorial, as well as information to help you write a script for finding your voice will be sent to you, by sending a request to the wondersofyoullc@gmail.com.

Questions/Comments: I would love to hear feedback from you! If you have any questions/comments about the book or anything that has been discussed, please email me at: thewondersofyoullc@gmail.com

Much love to you as you continue your journey!

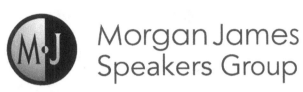

Morgan James
Speakers Group

www.TheMorganJamesSpeakersGroup.com

We connect Morgan James published
authors with live and online events
and audiences who will benefit
from their expertise.

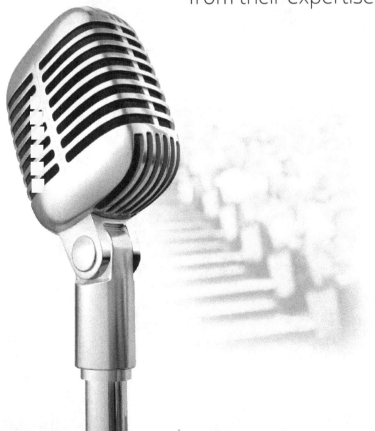

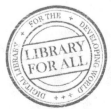